VEGAN KETO

*The Diet Everyone is Talking About
but No One Knows How to Do*

TAY SWEAT

ISBN: 978-1-7918-3943-7

Dedication

THIS BOOK, the how-to guide to vegan keto, is dedicated to all of those vegans out there who have been eating fruits and vegetables, trying to lose weight, and have been unsuccessful. You know who I'm talking about. The people who think they're following what's right but don't know that they're either insulin resistant or the PCOS they're dealing with or suffering from is the same thing that's is holding them back from losing the weight they are trying to lose.

This book is also dedicated to all of those non-vegans out there who are also doing the keto diet and who told us that vegan keto is impossible, that vegans just have to do high carbs.

This book is also dedicated to all of the other naysayers I was not able to cover. This is my attempt to show the world that not only can you be vegan, but you can also be vegan and low carb, while achieving the goals you have put forth, such as recovering from or improving PCOS, recovering or improving insulin resistance, or losing the weight that's been sticking around with you for years.

Also, to those of you who are diabetics, those of you who are maybe dealing with cognitive function issues, and those of you who may be dealing with hormone imbalance issues, this book is for you, too.

CONTENTS

TAY SWEAT

Introduction

IN THIS BOOK, I want to put to rest many of the questions vegans get and many of the crazy looks we receive when we tell someone, "Hey, I'm vegan, but I'm also keto."

You know what I'm talking about. You've probably told someone that you want to try out this diet or that you are already doing the diet, and some of the reactions you may get are:

"Plant-based keto? Vegan keto? Is that possible?"

"How are you getting your fats in? I thought vegan just meant you had to eat a bunch of carbs."

"It's not healthy to eat that many fats. Are you going to get fatty liver disease?"

"Aren't you going to hurt yourself by being so restrictive?"

"Doesn't it get boring?"

Okay, I'm sure you get it by now.

There are so many questions we get when it comes to the vegan keto diet, and that in itself is one of the reasons why I wrote this book, because I want to answer all the questions we hear, and I want to empower you, the reader, with the correct tool. Not only to be successful with the vegan keto diet, but to arm yourself with the proper information to combat some of these questions that you, too, may be getting from your friends, your family, your coworkers, and any other strangers on the street who may just be asking you how you eat.

The reason why I think this is important is because, once you go through and complete a full phase of a ketogenic, vegan, plant-based diet, you're going to lose a lot of fat. If you have PCOS, you're going to notice that your polycystic ovary syndrome (PCOS) gets better. If you have skin issues, you're going to notice that your skin is going to clear up. If you're dealing with insulin resistance or diabetes, that's going to get better, as well.

So, you're going to be walking around feeling and looking better, and people are going to know what you did to get these types of results. Therefore, it's my job not only to teach you how to get these results but also is to teach you how to respond to people when they ask you what it is you're doing, because many of us don't know how to explain a vegan ketogenic diet, let alone how to follow a proper vegan plant-based ketogenic diet.

Now, you may hear me talk in this book about "plant-based" very frequently. The reason is because I want to emphasize that the differences between vegan and plant-based are real.

What do I mean by that? When someone eats vegan, this usually means, as long as it's not an animal product, you can eat it. That means, if it does not include animal products, you can eat it, and it's vegan.

If you're walking down the street and you see an Oreo cookie on the ground, there aren't any animal products in that Oreo cookie. You can eat it. However, this may not be very healthy and may not serve you well in your health journey or even your weight-loss journey, for that matter.

But when it comes to plant-based, this word means that you exclusively eat plants. That doesn't mean cookies that are vegan, but it does mean that you cannot eat a bunch of processed foods.

Why is it important to stay away from processed foods? Well, let's just keep it real here. A processed food in its simplest form is a bowel movement. That's right. Poop, feces, shit—that's exactly what processed food is. Now, follow where I'm going here.

When we eat a natural food, a plant-based, whole food—notice the emphasis on the *whole*—our body starts to process this whole food by chewing.

Saliva mixes in with the food you are chewing and then you swallow, which starts the digestive system. In the digestive phase, you start to break down this food. This whole food that you ate has now been chewed, saliva added, and now it's starting to be separated. The body separates the nutrients you need from the food. The things you can use are pulled apart from the not-so-good things that are within this whole food.

Then, your body is going to utilize what's needed, or the productive part of the food, and it's going to poop out or release the food that it doesn't want or cannot use. This end product, the food it could not use or that has no nutritional value left for you in the body, this food that's being pooped out, is considered the processed food. It's the remains. The remaining product of the whole food you just ate.

If I take a whole grain—let's just say wheat, for example—and I send it through a "process" in some type of factory, I'm going to break down the wheat. I might bleach it. I might grind it up and pull out the things that are going to make this wheat go bad, if I leave it out on the shelf, so there goes all the enzymes the wheat might've had. I'm going to heat this wheat as high as possible, and I'm going to pulverize it until it's made into a powder. So now, we have bleached wheat that has been heated very high, processed, and turned into what you know as bleached white flour.

This bleached white flour is not a whole food. This bleached white flour is a processed food. All of the good things have been taken out of it. It's been heated, and now you are left over with the byproducts or the poop.

This is why we stay away from processed foods. First of all, because they're not so good for the body. Second of all, because we don't eat poop. We don't eat poop. *We don't eat poop.* (Just in case you needed to hear it three times.)

My goal with this book is to be as simple and clear as possible. We have way too many doctors and "smart people" who aim to use all of the big, million-dollar words that go over most of our heads, correct? Well, my goal is to be the opposite of that. Yes, I'm going to give you factual content. I'm going to give you content that has worked for thousands of my clients. I'm going to give you actual, factual content that has worked for me. However, I'm going to simplify most of this, so you're not constantly going to look up words like "gluconeogenesis" or "pollicis."

My goal is to simply make this book so easy to read that you can hand it to your three-year-old or four-year-old and they can understand exactly what I'm trying to say. Hopefully, they, too, can make sense out of a vegan plant-based keto diet, just like you can.

Chapter One

My Journey with Vegan Keto

I WANT TO GIVE you a little backstory about what I had to go through, where I come from, and how I eventually found my way to a plant-based vegan keto diet.

I was raised by a single mother of two boys in what's considered to be poverty. We didn't have a lot of money. We didn't have a lot of access to things. We went to inner-city schools, so we didn't know much about nutrition. We didn't know what a calorie was. We didn't know what a fat, carb, or protein was. As a matter of fact, just to be quite frank, we were just happy to be able to eat whenever we had food available.

Over time, this caused me to gain over 120 pounds, resulting in a 312-pound fifteen-year-old. Yes, I was athletic. Yes, I was very active. As a matter of fact, I was not one of the kids who played video games. My brother and I had to be outside, active, jumping on trampolines, playing basketball, or running around the neighborhood. I was always active in sports throughout my childhood, even during and after the weight gain.

However, with all of this activity and lots of sports activities my mom had us signed up for, my mom was doing a lot of taxi work. She was driving from one side of the city to the other to be at games or school events. This resulted in my mom being stretched for time, including not having time to cook. So, on the fly, Mom would just stop and get us miscellaneous restaurant food, okay? Fast food.

A lot of this fast food resulted in me gaining this weight. I didn't realize I was gaining that much weight until I reached my highest weight, 312 pounds. It was then that people started to call me names. People started to look at me weird. Even when I played basketball, people would look at me and ask why was I on the court? "You're too fat to play basketball," they'd say.

Through this weight gain, I also started to generate other issues in my body, such as high blood pressure, childhood or juvenile diabetes-type 2, eczema, and heart disease. These things seemed like they came out of nowhere. This was when I took my life into my own hands and realized, if I didn't do something about the weight, I was going to die an early death.

It was then that I started to do my research and my studies on different foods, on what a calorie was, what a fat was, what a protein and what a carb were. Upon doing all of this studying—mind you, I was only about sixteen—I started to carry water around. I started to look different. I stood out. I was the only teenager in my high school carrying around a gallon of water. I was the only teenager in my high school eating a salad for lunch. While all the other kids were eating French fries, pizza, and donuts, I was eating salad and water. That's right. I was very healthy, considering where I came from.

This paid off, because, over an eighteen-month period, I lost over 120 pounds. I made it to a weight that looked acceptable for my height at the time. And now people were wondering, what did I do? How did I lose weight so fast?

One of the secrets to my success was the simple fact that I stopped eating a lot of the processed foods. There was no more McDonald's. There was no more Jack in the Box. There were no more fast food windows, period.

Not only that, through the studying I was doing over the course of that eighteen months, I saw I should probably be eating more vegetables, more fruits, and, of course, I should be getting my protein. But through this journey, I also noted that the more I could eliminate from my diet, the better and faster I could lose the weight.

So I did that. I lost the weight. Everything was great. However, I did not keep it off. Why? Because I was doing a lot of binge eating and intermittent fasting. I took that to the next level and wouldn't eat for days, but then I would go around playing basketball, totally fasted, and then binge eat afterward.

Now, most of you are going to say, "Well, why would I fast?" This is something we'll talk about more in this book. But it's not the fasting that got me. It was the binge eating that got me. I mention this simply because I want you to know that while some of you likely are fasting right now, you're not getting the results, because you are binge eating after you come out of the fast. That is what we have to avoid and be careful of.

So, years go by. I'm now an adult, and I still have yet to get rid of my diabetes, my insulin resistance, my heart disease, and my eczema. What's going on? I decide to further my studies.

I started to go out and get certifications on how to do certain things. I really put a lot of time into getting healthy, because I really wanted to get rid of some of these things. Based on my studies up to this point in my life, I'd seen that these things could be improved or reversed through proper nutrition. So, I started to eliminate things and noticed that, hey, a vegetarian diet is the way to go. Let's try it out.

But, upon my trying out a vegetarian diet, whenever I shared it with family, friends, and people I thought were concerned about my health, these people told me, "Well, be careful, because that's a dangerous diet. Where are you going to get your protein from? Where are you going to get your vitamins from?"

Now, up until then, nobody was a nutritionist. Nobody had any information to help me lose the weight. But when I told them I was now going to try out a vegan diet, suddenly everybody knew so much. And of course, my first thought was, "Where were you all when I needed you the most? Where was this information?"

Of course, I got no answers to that, so I just continued to do my self-studies, keeping in mind all of the concerns they had for me, such as protein.

Throughout this journey, I slowly began to eliminate meats from my diet, starting with red meat, and then going down to chicken, turkey, and eventually getting rid of all meat and eating only fish. Then, eventually, I got rid of the fish, too. So then I was only eating a little dairy, plus vegetables, lots of nuts and seeds, and, of course, a few fruits.

Because I was told I needed to watch for protein, most of my nutrition, or most of my calories, were coming from nuts and seeds at this time. I was making very big smoothies with lots of nuts and seeds, plus coconut milk—really trying to get in the protein. Little did I know I didn't need as much as I was attempting to get, but I kept trying and trying. I would eat a lot of nuts and seeds, and I would follow that up with avocado and vegetables. And, of course, I would have a little fruit, but not too much, because they tell you, "Don't have too much sugar."

So, I listened to some of these "nutritionists" who'd been hiding when I needed them the most. I watched my sugar, I made sure I got my protein, and I ate my veggies like my mom taught me to. What this birthed was—although I had no idea it was at the time—a small version of a keto diet.

Yes, that's right. Before ketogenic diets were even in existence as a marketing ploy or something with a label, I was doing it, and I had no idea I was doing it. I was eating nuts. I was eating seeds. I was eating lots of fatty fruits, like avocados and olives, because I love olives. The keto diet was in my life, and I had no idea I was doing it.

This resulted in, one, my losing the weight I'd gained back, because I'd gained about fifty pounds of the initial weight I lost—I got that fifty pounds back off, plus some. Two, I finally had abs now, so I was rocking the six pack. Not only that, the eczema finally went away. The diabetes was gone. The heart disease was nonexistent. The hypertension gone. And yes, at this point, I was still practicing fasting, but I was no longer binging. I was doing everything more strategically. I was also doing it around my working schedule, because I was a man now, and I had to work.

Now, it wasn't until six or seven years later that I realized a vegan keto diet is exactly what I was doing. I was just simply trying to follow the advice from all of the "nutritionists" who were giving me their hidden wisdom.

Years go by, and I'm now telling people I'm vegan, because I no longer eat dairy or eggs. But when I tell people I'm vegan, of course they look at my diet and ask, "Where's your fruit? You should be able to eat a high-carbohydrate diet and get away with it. Why aren't you eating rice and grains and beans? Why are you not eating that?"

There weren't many vegans around at this point, so I didn't want to appear weird to my newfound vegan friends. I joined the club. I started to eat a diet high in fruits and high in grains, along with high amounts of beans. I basically switched to a high-carbohydrate diet. Little did I know this doesn't work well with my body.

These changes resulted in my storing a little weight around my gut and stomach area. It also resulted in my gaining a little more weight on the scale. And, to be honest, I really didn't feel as well.

So, what did I have to do? I started testing things out. I worked on a raw vegan diet that consisted of only fruits and slightly steamed vegetables. That diet went very well. I lost a lot of fat, but I lost a lot of muscle, as well. That diet was the cleanest diet I'd ever eaten, because I didn't eat anything cooked. It was all raw or lightly steamed. And I did feel good on the diet.

Would I recommend it to people who are interested in that type of thing? Absolutely. But if you are someone who wants the butt and the thighs, if you want a nice build, you want arms, you want a nice chest, and you want to build some big muscle, would I suggest that diet? Probably not. Maybe a refinement of that diet, where we add in some other things, but that's a story for another book.

If you are someone who wants to get those butt muscles and those sculpted thighs, if you want the arms, fellas, and you want the back and the biceps, the chest and the shoulders, if you want to maintain or grow these, while also leaning out and getting the abs and cutting fat, the keto diet stands as the number one choice for me.

Around this time, I was now training other clients. I'm certified in over five different subjects. Now I'm starting to apply the keto diet, the vegan plant-based keto diet, to many of my clients.

Chapter Two

What is Vegan Ketosis and How Do We Get to that State?

KETOSIS IS A STATE of burning ketones for fuel by way of burning or using fat as energy.

What does that mean? Many people are glucose or sugar burners, which means you eat carbohydrates. And, by default, you burn glucose as your main source of energy. Up until maybe the last decade or two, this was the only way the mainstream media knew how to describe how we live. This was the only way. And if you did anything outside of that, you were going to hurt yourself or you were not in an ideal eating pattern or ideal eating state.

But the new research that has come out in the last decade or two is showing that being fat-fueled is much more efficient and effective. And we live is metabolic flexibility, which is basically being able to burn *both* glucose from carbohydrates *and* ketones from burning fat.

To sum it up, ketosis is a state where you're going to be running on fat for your fuel or for your energy. This fat produces an exhaust-like byproduct called ketones. And this is what many people have been using to fix, repair, and even reverse some things like PCOS, or type-two diabetes. They can also improve type-one diabetes, by minimizing the insulin response from the foods we eat. Weight loss has been huge with this diet or approach. In addition to that, hormone optimization has been definitely improved.

Now, let's dive into how to get into ketosis.

Many of you have probably heard of intermittent fasting. It's all over the Internet. It's all over the blogs. All of the influencers are doing it. Everyone on YouTube seems to want to talk about it. It's a hot topic. But what is it, really? And why are so many people using intermittent fasting?

Well, in short, intermittent fasting is a time-restrictive way of eating. Intermittent fasting basically calls for you to put yourself in a window of eating, to eat only within a given amount of time. Anything outside of that, you will refrain from food or consuming calories overall.

What does an intermittent fast look like? How can you make this work for you, in your lifestyle? How can this help you to get into ketosis faster? And how can this help you with your goals and your overall journey?

Well, intermittent fasting is very, very, very simple. It is very efficient and effective because many people in this day and age don't have the time, the scheduling, or even the patience to eat every two to three hours, like your average bodybuilding or personal training coach wants you to do.

Intermittent fasting is something that the everyday person thrives on, because guess what? You don't have to wake up and eat breakfast. And then guess what? If you're stuck in traffic or you have to get your kids to school or you have some important meeting, you don't have to rush to eat your next snack after breakfast.

And guess what? If you're still busy and you're still on the go or you still have some work to do and you still can't get to some food, you still don't have to eat at lunch. You can go right past lunch.

I personally fast anywhere from between eighteen and twenty-three hours on most days. It's very efficient. It works well for me as an entrepreneur. It works well for me as a husband, and it works well for me as an overall man.

Because it allows me to get work done. It allows me to spread myself across, so I have balance in my life, while still maintaining a very, very efficient diet.

I don't have to eat something on the go and just settle for any type of food, just because I need a meal. I have the opportunity now to eat when the time is right and when the actual environment allows for me to eat.

What does that mean? Many people fall prey to eating fast food, junk food, or processed food. Remember we talked about not eating processed food?

Well, many people are having to settle for processed foods, because that is all that's available at the time.

When I go through airports, I see so many people having to settle for airport food. Why? Because they have to eat. They have to get their energy, right? They have to have some sustenance for the plane ride, correct? Not correct. No.

When you practice intermittent fasting, when you get good and when you get ideally fat-adapted, you can bypass all of the airport foods. You can bypass all of the processed foods that are sitting around, waiting on you to purchase them. The fast food restaurants—you can bypass all of these things.

Why? Because when you become fat-adapted and you practice intermittent fasting, so you are now using your internal energy or your "stored fat," "stored energy." You are using that now for your energy source.

So, for those of you who say, "Well, I have to eat to get energy," not anymore. Intermittent fasting is the way to get away from that. And I'm going to show you how you can implement it into your own life.

Let's just start with the normal average day, based on the average client I see in my practice. A client comes in and lets me know they usually sleep for about six to seven hours. We'll say six, because most people are only getting six hours. From there, they wake up, and they're off to the races. They either have kids to attend to, or they have an early meeting, or they have to work out. There's always something in the morning that gets in the way of eating breakfast, and that's okay.

Then this person goes through the rest of their day busy, of course, because we're all busy in our own way. And by the end of the day, this person has eaten very little. As a matter of fact, they're ready to binge on food at dinnertime.

This binge comes, of course, from not completing or not doing a proper intermittent fasting protocol. So now, your insulin levels are high (insulin levels being elevated are very much responsible for the cravings you have later on in the day). So, if you make it through a day, say you had a little snack and then you didn't eat anything in between, by the time dinner time is here, you are craving all types of foods. And this is where many people get in trouble on their weight-loss journey or on their health journey overall.

What am I saying here? Basically, if you're going to snack in the morning or if you're going to have something in the morning and you want to eat later on for dinner, then more than likely the program you need to follow is more of a "every two to three hours" type of program. That means you should eat at 6:00 AM. You should eat at 10:00 AM. You should eat at noon. You should eat at 3:00 PM. And you should eat at 6:00 PM. This is your eating schedule. Why? Because this is one of the natural ways of feeding the human body.

How do we know this? If you do your research on the feeding process during human gestation, the child or the fetus is fed in this fashion. When a woman is pregnant, she is providing nutrients to the child at 6:00 AM with a big amount of nutrients. At 10:00 AM, she feeds the child a snack. At noon, there's another big feeding. At 3:00 PM, the woman is now feeding the child a light snack. And then at 6:00 PM, the child eats another heavy serving of nutrients, and that's it for the day.

If you want to do that little snacking throughout the day, you can't have it both ways. You can't eat one snack and then fast, and then eat again for dinner. This is what causes your insulin levels to stay high, and this is what also causes you to crave many things you shouldn't be eating. This is what messes people up. If you're going to go for an extended period without eating, do not break your fast. Just go ahead and go through that period without food until you can get to your food.

So, those are your two options. You may eat throughout the day, or you may fast until you can eat something that is in alignment with your nutrition and health goals. This time, let's take the same client's schedule, and apply intermittent fasting.

Let's say you are the average person who sleeps about six hours a night, and let's say that you want to be a healthy person, so you stop eating the recommended three hours before bed. This is already a nine hour fast. You stop eating three hours before bed, and you sleep six hours, so you are now nine hours fasting. It feels good, right? Many people don't think about it, but this is a part of your fast.

Then you wake up, let's just say at 6:00 AM. You wake up, and you skip breakfast because you're busy. You don't have time to make breakfast, not for yourself. Maybe for your kids, but not for yourself. Not a healthy breakfast at that. So, you make the kids breakfast or you get to your meeting, or you get to the gym or you get where you need to go. You get the day running, you get the day started by skipping breakfast.

Before you know it, you're at lunchtime. You've gone from 6:00 AM to lunchtime at noon, 12:00 PM. Which is another six hours. You, my friend, have now fasted for fifteen hours.

This is exactly what the recommended window is for the average person. Finish food three hours before bed, sleep for six or seven hours, and don't eat until lunchtime. This is intermittent fasting. This is your most practical and popular form of doing intermittent fasting, which is called the 16/8. You go about sixteen hours without food, and you eat within an eight-hour window.

Now, where can we find this in nature? We're going to go to the circadian rhythm for this one. As most of you know, we have twenty-four hours in a day, and we humans on this planet who live through those twenty-four hours also have a twenty-four-hour clock called the circadian rhythm. This circadian rhythm is broken down into three eight-hour windows.

Each window's time is associated with an act or a system of actions. What that means is you have the first eight-hour window, starting around 3:00 AM and going to about 11:00 AM. This window is what we call the purging period. I'm going to start here because this is the most important to me.

The purging period is when we take nutrients. The purging period is when our body takes all the waste from the things it can't use and doesn't want from the previous day or the previous week or the previous year (because some of you are full of waste that the body is still trying to get rid of from years ago), and the body, during this purging period, deals with this waste it is trying to get rid of. That is why, when you wake up in the morning, you usually pee and poop, or at least you should.

This is the body saying, "Hey, it's time to get rid of whatever we have been doing and don't need from the past days."

And I know what you're thinking. "But breakfast is the most important meal of the day, right? So why aren't we eating?"

Well, you are not wrong. Breakfast is the most important meal of the day. However, breakfast is a combination of two words. "Break" and "fast." Breakfast. And break fast or breaking your fast is the most important meal of the day because it is important that you eventually break your fast. However, we do not break our fast in most cases until 11:00, maybe even noon. The reason why is because the second eight-hour window within this twenty-four hours starts around 11 AM or maybe even high noon.

You may know it to be noon or lunchtime, and it goes up until about 7:00 PM to maybe even 8:00 PM. The reason why I'm giving you these ranges is because, of course, we have time changes. We have people who shift through different time zones, whether you're traveling for work or moving to a new area.

This second eight-hour window is the feeding window. This is the time when your body is primed to eat its nutrients and everything it can for the day. Why? Because this is the time when the body actually wants to take the nutrients in and use them, start to break the food down. So, this is when you eat. And with us being "sun people" or people of the sun, of course we get a lot of our energy and nutrients from the sun.

The sun also gives us extra energy to digest foods, which is why we start eating when the sun is at its highest point. That is why I also said high noon, because high noon is a perfect time for the body to start eating and utilizing nutrients.

So, let's go into our third eight-hour window, which starts around 8:00 PM. Now, this eight-hour window is the utilization phase. During this phase, this is where the body is taking the foods you just ate and starts to utilize and break them down.

What does that mean? If you ate something that was fifty percent nutritious and good and usable for the body, and if the other fifty percent was crap and the body can't do anything with it, what this phase is for is to break down that food, send the fifty percent where it needs to go, and then, of course, it's going to send the other fifty percent—the junk—over to the colon to be purged during the next eight-hour window.

So, once you have completed the full twenty-four hours and gone through a purging phase, an eating phase, and a utilization phase, it just starts over again the next day.

Now, if you fast for twenty hours and you only have a four-hour eating window, then you can just pick four hours within that 12 to 8:00 PM window. If you want to go a full twenty-four hours, that's fine. Make sure you break your fast inside of that same window.

Once again, this is what I do for myself. This is what I do for my clients. The science proves it. The biology of humanity proves it. This is what works. This is what has worked for us for years.

Now, I know what you thinking. How does this help me get into ketosis much faster? Well, during the fasting period or the period when you are refraining from eating, you will slowly start to rely on nutrients that are inside of your body.

Let's say you start with a sixteen-hour fast. The body is going to start using up things that are in the body, the stored energy. And, of course, this is why we want to fast, because we want the body to become accustomed to using this stored energy or what you call fat. If you fast for these sixteen hours, the body has to get energy from somewhere, correct? This is what starts the process of getting into ketosis.

Now, let's be honest with ourselves here. Sixteen hours is not enough time to go through the stored nutrients that you have, which is called glycogen. Okay? For those of you who don't know, quick reference: glycogen is what the body stores in the liver and the muscles from carbohydrates you have eating. So, if you've been eating too many carbohydrates and your glycogen is full, you get what we call fat spillover. This fat spillover is one of the things that's responsible for the fat gain throughout the year.

It is important to note that it takes up to twenty-four hours or maybe even longer to properly or fully drain the muscle glycogen or drain the liver glycogen to a point to where the body starts to feed or fuel itself on fats.

What does this mean? This means that although intermittent fasting can be helpful to slowly get you into ketosis, it is not the fastest way and not the most efficient way of doing it. This is where of course we get into the three-day extended fast.

Now, I know what you thinking. Why would anybody go three days without food?

To start, it's therapeutic. A three-day fast is very helpful to the body, because it can help to reset your systems. It can reset your immune system. It can regenerate dead cells or cells that weren't helpful. Not only that, it can help with things like atherosclerosis, which is a hardening of the arteries, the clogging up of the arteries after people have been eating a not-so-nutritious diet, leading to artery blockage and high blood pressure.

Some men even have erectile dysfunction. Some women have issues getting blood flow down to their genital area and are having dry vagina. Some people are having some type of issues with a wound due to lack of blood flow and nutrients to help it heal. A seventy-two-hour fast can help to eat away at some of these things, like the plaque that is blocking blood flow and causing many of these issues.

But what else can a three-day fast do, and why is it so important in getting us into ketosis?

Well, the intermittent fasting protocol works great, but the three-day fast has much more powerful ways of getting the job done, simply because the first twenty-four hours are only going to be dedicated to muscle and liver glycogen. You're only going to use the stored carbohydrates that you have. So, if you're only doing twenty-four or maybe thirty-six hours of fasting, your body is only going to use the carbohydrates that you have stored. When you go back and eat, you're just going to re-store carbohydrates. You never get to burn fat in that scenario.

However, if you do a three-day fast, the first twenty-four to thirty-six hours is going to be dedicated to burning through those carbohydrates that have been stored. We call it glycogen. But during the next few hours, after the twenty-four to thirty-six, you start to burn fat. This is called lipolysis, for those of you want to go do your research on that. Now, at this point, the body starts to break down fat cells and use them for energy.

This is where it gets important, because the body is now becoming accustomed to burning fat. Before now, it was only burning carbs and glycogen. Glucose. Which means, if you're only burning glucose, later on when you start giving the body more fat, the body is not going to accept it, which I will talk about a little bit later.

So now you're in the thirty-six- to forty-eight-hour window, and you're burning lots of good fat. This is the time where you're also starting to produce ketones, because when we burn fat, the byproduct or the exhaust byproduct from burning fat is ketone bodies. Now the body is getting accustomed to burning fat and using ketones. This is how we slingshot—that's what I call it— this is how we slingshot our way into ketosis, without getting the keto from other things.

Now, after the forty-eight hours, your body will slowly start to go into what we call autophagy. Autophagy literally means cellular death or the death of cells. You are going to now not only burn fat cells, but the body is also going to start burning not-so-good cells. So, if you have some cancer cells running around in the body, a three-day fast has been proven in studies to utilize and burn-up cancerous cells. Also, other cells that may be just dormant or junk cells. So, this three-day fast going to help you start to burn through those cells and really get things cleaned up. Cleaning up the house.

You may also be worried about losing protein, because you've heard that a seventy-two-hour or three-day fast also starts to utilize protein. We don't want to lose our good, hard-earned muscle.

Well, I'm here to tell you that you will not be losing your hard-earned muscle during the burning of protein. Why? Because the body, at this point, is burning protein from things like extra skin. Things like extra cells inside the body that aren't useful. Once again, autophagy.

This has been huge not only for me but for a lot of my clients who have a lot of weight to lose. Because this skin I am referring to is the skin we have leftover when we lose a lot of weight. So, when I lost 120 pounds, one of the biggest reasons why my body was able to adjust and not have a lot of sagging skin was because I did a lot of fasting through my weight-loss journey. And this fasting, of course, started to utilize proteins, and the proteins came from that extra skin and other extra cells that weren't useful to my body.

Now, if this doesn't make sense for you, I have a pretty cool—I like to think it's cool—story or analogy that I like to use. And that is basically a sinking ship.

When your body goes into a fast, you can consider it to be a sinking ship. And in a sinking ship, it's only sinking because it's heavy. So, what are we going to get rid of? If the body is sinking like a sinking ship, does it get rid of the engine and the gas and the steering wheel, all of the things that are helping it to power forward and be great? Are we going to get rid of those things while the ship is sinking? No. Our body is no different. The body's not going to get rid of its engine, its origins, its muscles.

It's not going to get rid of the good stuff it needs to survive. It needs to thrive, so that's not how the body works. The body is actually going to get rid of things like junk.

Some of the things on the ship that are considered junk may be trash. We likely have trash piled up from dinners on previous nights and other waste. We're going to start throwing that off the ship, so we don't sink. We're trying to make the boat lighter, so we don't sink.

We're also going to start throwing things off that we don't need, like tables and chairs. We don't necessarily need tables and chairs on this ship, not if we're trying to stay alive. So, let's get rid of some of these tables and chairs so we can stay alive. Let's get rid of the waste, the trash, and all of this stuff we don't need or use on this ship. Let's get rid of it. Let's throw it off the ship, so the ship can stay afloat. We *can* get light enough so we don't sink.

That's exactly what the body does. It gets rid of the waste. It gets rid of all of the liquid manure, the liquid poop. (You hear me talk about that a lot.) It gets rid of the waste while you're fasting. Because, once again, the average person has up to fifteen to thirty pounds of waste or liquid manure poop in their body. You may know it to be called plaque or mucoid plaque, but the body has up to fifteen to thirty pounds of this waste, mucoid plaque or poop in the body. So, when the body goes through a fast, it's going to utilize that first. It's not going after your precious muscle. I can guarantee you that.

After you complete this seventy-two-hour fast, you didn't lose any muscle. You lost glycogen, you lost a little fat. And if you were doing a little cardio, say a little walking (which is pretty much the only cardio I suggest during a three-day fast) during this period, you probably lost more fat than the average person will.

But the big thing here is your body is now familiar with burning fats. So now, it starts to burn fats for fuel. When I give you a diet full of high-fat food now, your body knows how to burn this high-fat food.

Now, why is this important? Because if we didn't go through this state of teaching and forcing the body to burn fat by way of a three-day fast, then the body may not accept a higher fat diet, simply because you've been feeding your face plenty of carbohydrates for ten, twenty, thirty, forty, fifty years. What happens is your body, in essence, forgets how to burn fat for fuel, which is why you're probably holding onto fat right now. It doesn't want to use fat for fuel.

In many cases, when people bypass this fasting period or decide not to fast because they just want to jump directly into a high-fat diet. What often happens next is that they get gag reflexes. Their body tries to reject all of the fat you're eating. In the simplest form, your body is saying, basically, "Hey, I'm not using the fat you have in your stomach. Why are you trying to give me fat from an outside source? You've been giving me carbs, and that's where I get my energy. So, I only want carbs. I am going to throw up or try to reject any excess fatty foods you eat."

This has happened to me and my clients when we try to bypass the fasting period. It's very important.

However, when we go through the fasting phase, we get into ketosis through fasting. The body then says, "Okay, we're going to use fat as fuel. I think I remember how to do this thing." It burns through the fats and then, when you give it fat after you break your fast, it knows what to do with it, because it just got done utilizing fat specifically.

This is huge, if you want to do a ketosis diet or a vegan keto diet.

Now, how do you break your fast? I'm sure that's what you're asking now. The best way to break your fast is with a high fatty fruit. One is an avocado. Two, you can also eat olives. Now, let's just say you don't want to break your fast with fruit. You'd rather have vegetables. I personally suggest and like to eat fermented vegetables to break a fast. Why? Because they are probiotics, and you can find a lot of great nutrients inside these fermented veggies.

Of course, this is if you want to stay in ketosis. A lot of you are probably thinking, "Well, I thought we're supposed to be eating other fruits and berries to break a fast."

These foods may not necessarily serve you the best, because they may kick you out of ketosis. So, I always suggest eating a high-fat fruit or some fermented veggies like sauerkraut or fermented cabbage and beets.

This has worked wonders for me and many others. Now, let's just say you don't want to do a three-day fast. That's a little too hardcore for you. Maybe it just doesn't sound like something you can do. Maybe you have some important things to do tomorrow and can't do a three-day fast. What's your other option?

Well, of course, one option is to not do any fasting and try to eat your way into ketosis. But I have to warn you: I have seen this take much longer to get into ketosis, which means you're going to struggle getting there. Not only that, you run the risk of getting keto flu, keto rash, and many of the other keto issues that come with doing it incorrectly.

Also, this process can last anywhere from two weeks to six months. I've seen it go as long as six months with some clients. With that being said, I would either do the three-day fast to slingshot or speed up the process of getting into ketosis.

Another alternative is called a fasting-mimicking diet. The fasting-mimicking diet was created and has been made popular by the doctor, Valter Longo. Valter Longo has studied at USC and done very, very intricate studies around fasting and the fasting-mimicking diet.

The fasting-mimicking diet is a five-day-only eating plan that you do maybe once a month or twice a year. You can do it quarterly, or every other month. It's totally up to you how you want to do it, but it's only for five days at a time. This is what it looks like.

On day one of the five days, you do a lower-calorie diet, in the range of 800 to 1100 calories. Then, on days two through five, you do an even lower-calorie range, eating between 500 and 750 calories.

I challenge you to go and do research with Dr. Valter Longo. Go to his page, Google him. Go check out his information, if you want to do this diet. I am simply referencing another option that you may use. But because this is not something I use inside of my nutrition planning for my clients, I'm going to refer you to Dr. Valter Longo or his web page, so you can get his research straight from the guy himself.

Although the fasting-mimicking diet works to help you get into ketosis, I don't use it because I like the fasting benefits much better. I find them to be more profound, plus it happens much quicker. That is why we use a three-day fast or intermittent fasting over the fasting-mimicking diet.

To end this chapter, you're probably thinking, "So I have to fast either way, to get into ketosis?"

No, you don't. You really don't. But once again, you run the risk of the process taking much longer. You run the risk of also possibly getting keto flu, keto rash, and other things, simply because your body has been used to burning carbohydrates for so long, it doesn't or won't want the fats you are going to try to give it.

So, take a quick examination of yourself and your situation, your schedule, and your life. Ask yourself, "Can I sneak in a three-day fast? Or should I do something like a fasting-mimicking diet? Or should I just try to eat my way into ketosis?"

Either way will work, but of course there are better ways of doing it based on the individual.

Chapter Three

Things to Look for Now that You Are in Ketosis

NOW YOU'VE DONE your fasting. You've done what it takes to get your body into ketosis. You're eating the proper fats, carbs, proteins, and calories for your body. So what should you look for now?

This is the chapter where we're going to talk about how much should you be eating, how to test for ketones, the types of ketones you need to be looking for, and much more.

Macros. The biggest question I get is, "What macros should I be following?"

Macros are basically protein, carbs, and fats. Macro is short for macronutrients. We have micronutrients, too, which are your minerals and your vitamins, and we have macronutrients, which are your protein, carbs, fats, and ketones. Ketones are considered the fourth macronutrient. Alcohol is also considered a macronutrient. These things are basically what we want to take into play, when it comes to dealing with your keto diet.

Usually, most people go to the Internet and look for traditional keto macros, which are usually seventy to eighty percent fat, with twenty to thirty percent from protein. Yes, I have seen it that high.

Now, of course, this is a meat-based philosophy that can work for a plant-based diet. However, from my personal experience, with my own body and the experience with hundreds of my clients, we've come to realize that these macros aren't sustainable. They don't necessarily work for us vegans. The simple reason that is because, in essence, to follow something like this, we basically have to limit our vegetables. And to be honest, as a nutrition coach, as a trainer and as a holistic practitioner, I don't like the sound of limiting vegetables.

So, we eat our vegetables, and we eat them in abundance. Of course, I'm not here to tell you exactly which macro ratio you should follow. I'm simply here to let you know what works for me, what has worked for hundreds of my clients, and what continues to work for many other people. This is what we call testing and tweaking.

Testing and tweaking your diet or your macros is based on your testing and tweaking your ketones. If you want to start with intermittent fasting or, what I suggest, a three-day fast, you will automatically be in ketosis with the three-day fast. From here, you test your ketones.

After your fast, you want to test your blood ketones to see where you are. If you don't know, the international standard way of measuring ketone and blood glucose levels is in terms of a molar concentration, measured in Mmol/L (millimoles per liter; or millimolar, abbreviated Mmol). From .5 millimolars up to 5.0 millimolars, you are considered to be in nutritional ketosis. Anything under .5 Mmol, you're not in ketosis, and anything over 5.0 Mmol, you are probably producing too many ketones and need to backup.

Now, check where you are in your testing after the three-day fast. Many people will be at 2.0 Mmol, 3.0 Mmol, sometimes even 4.0 millimolars, and that's okay. This is not a game I want you to get obsessed with, playing to see how many ketones or who has the highest number of ketones produced. It's all totally fine.

It's totally fine so long as you are in nutritional ketosis. So yes, I am saying, if you're only producing or you only have .5 on the millimolar test, you are in ketosis. You are good. As someone who may be producing 3.0 Mmol, it's totally fine. Don't get caught up in playing this game, because I've seen people get hurt this way.

Now, go into your diet with the starting point of ketones or macros you would like to start with. So, for instance, if you wanted to start with seventy or eight percent, for instance—say 70% from fat, 20% from protein, 10% from carbs—then go into this one first. You want to start with this macro breakdown and test. What do your ketones look like a day after? What do your ketones look like two days after?

What happens is, if you notice, you'll still have ketones in your blood and you're good to go. Maybe you can even start to up the ratios, meaning maybe you could start to add a few more carbohydrates from vegetables. Maybe you can start to lower the fat just a little bit. This is where we continue to tweak and test.

After you add a few more vegetables, what do your ketones look like now? What I usually suggest is that people continue to tweak and test until they kick themselves out of ketosis. As long as you can do this, you will be in a good state.

As soon as you kick yourself out of ketosis, you have to tweak back, which means you may have raised your calories or your carbs too high. When carbs have gone too high, it will kick you out of ketosis, and it's time to backpedal. Maybe you've eaten too much fruit or maybe you had too many vegetables. Whatever it is, now you're kicked out of ketosis and it's time to reverse that. It's time to start going back up in fat and down in carbohydrates.

Some of us have gotten away with eating more fruit than people would suggest. For instance, I've personally been able to eat upwards of 200 grams of carbs and get away with staying in ketosis. Of course, I'm an athlete. Many people wouldn't be able to do this.

I've also been able to do other things like this simply by tweaking and testing with my clients. I have some women doing 100 grams of carbs, for example, with of course many of them coming from vegetables. These are total carbs, by the way.

Side note: total carbs means the overall amount of carbohydrates you are eating. You will see, upon your research, many people say "net carbs." Net carbs are basically total carbs minus fiber. So, if we have 100 grams of total carbs and we have 40 grams of fiber, that means we're left with 60 grams of net carbs. This is how it works.

I'm here to show you how to do all of this and to explain all of this. With that being said, I also want to show you how to get your calories. Many of you are eating way too little or way too few overall calories. This is causing you metabolic damage, and it causes you to hold on to fat. It's also causing you to slow down in your results.

When you're doing a keto diet, you can actually eat a few more calories. What I suggest for someone who's looking to lose fat, say you want to lose more than ten or twenty pounds, multiply your body weight by ten. This is going to be the calorie range I want you to follow. From there, you're just going to it break down into 70% of these calories from fat, 20% of these calories from protein, and the last 10% of these calories from carbs.

Now, many of you are maybe going to get tripped up and start to think, "That's crazy! I don't know how to do any of this."

That's okay. You've got the Google machine. And, of course, you can always come to @iamthevegantrainer on Instagram and ask me any questions you may have. I'm here to help. I'm here to help you guide yourself. But I want you to be able to do this on your own, so you don't have to pay anybody.

Now, for people who are a little more active and just looking to slightly lose weight, less than fifteen or so pounds of weight or fat (I like to say *fat*, not just weight),

I want you to multiply your body weight times twelve. This will be your calorie range.

Anyone who's looking to maintain their body weight but wants to lose a little fat (so, basically, they want to build a little muscle but also lose the same amount of fat they gained in muscle), you're going to multiply your body weight by fifteen. Now, these are very generalized ways of calculating your estimated daily calories. There are other ways to do it, but I want to give you something simple.

If you are an athlete or you're looking to gain a lot of weight, so you want to gain muscle, or ladies, if you want to grow your butt and/or grow your thighs, but you're happy with your abs or with your stomach, then you want to multiply your body weight times eighteen to twenty. Twenty is going to be a little aggressive, but if you want to gain this weight pretty fast, I would do twenty. If you want to be a little more on the careful side, I would do eighteen.

Now that you have your calorie ranges and the percentages you're going to follow, let's go into how to test for your ketones, to see where you are.

First, I'm going to start off with the urine test. Many people are going to go buy the ketone sticks that call for you to urinate on the stick. This is only going to work for about two to four weeks. Usually, after that, your body stops peeing out ketones.

What do I mean by stops peeing out ketones? Similar to unwanted or unused vitamins that are released through your urine, ketones are also released through your urine when your body can't or doesn't want to use them. This ketone that's coming through your urine is called acetoacetate. With that being said, usually, when you're peeing out ketones, your body has not been adapted or has not adapted enough to use the ketones. So yes, it just urinates them out.

It's very smart for you to actually use this test for the first two to three weeks, stay on your keto diet, and then go into measuring blood ketones.

With blood testing, you are going to have to prick yourself. I know many of you hate to prick yourself to draw blood. However, this is one of the most efficient and accurate ways to test for ketones. The ketone body that's going to be in your blood is called beta-hydroxybutyrate. This blood ketone will let us know, one, that we're utilizing ketones, especially if they're not coming out of your urine anymore; and two, it's going to let us know where we are as far as the ketone scale. Of course, you want to be .5 Mmol or higher. This is the method I use to test my ketones. It works very effectively, and it's very accurate.

One machine I suggest you buy is the Keto-Mojo, M-O-J-O. The Keto-Mojo works very well. It's about $60, and it will get you your ketone strips, as well as your glucose strips, if you want to test glucose as well, which we will not be getting into in this book. And then next, of course, you want to make sure you have enough ketone strips. The Keto-Mojo is going to come with about fifty initially. After that, you'll have to re-supply your ketone strips.

If you are one of the people who doesn't necessarily like to test or prick yourself for the blood ketone test, then, we have the breath test. The breath ketone in the body is acetone. This ketone body is usually detected by the way your breath or your how spit/saliva tastes, and by the way your breath smells. You can almost always tell when you have acetone in your breath.

With this method, you are going to need to buy a ketone breathalyzer, which usually costs about $150 to $300. One breathalyzer brand you can check out is called Ketonix. It can be found on Amazon.com for $150-$300 bucks. You simply blow into this meter, and it gives you your results.

Next, you have your macros and your calories. You will know what to test for and how to adjust your macros based on the ketones you're pulling. But for now, we're going to talk about what you should be looking for.

A few things you're going to be looking for, are things like keto flu or symptoms of keto flu, which are basically symptoms of the normal flu. Your throat may feel a little scratchy or itchy. You may have a cough or a snotty, running nose. You may develop a fever.

You may also get what's called keto rash, where you'll have a rash appear on a given part of your body.

I've seen it on legs. I've seen on my arms. So, look out for that. You may also get breakouts on your face. This comes from doing keto incorrectly wrong. These few things come from not having the proper electrolytes, magnesium, potassium, and, of course, iodine in your diet.

What my clients use to avoid this is called Magic Moss. That's right: if you have been following me for a while, you've heard or seen me taking Magic Moss before and after my gym workouts. You have seen me taking Magic Moss before bed, too. You have seen me taking Magic Moss during my fasting times and also during those times when I need my minerals like magnesium, potassium, and iodine.

Magic Moss is made up of a combination of sea vegetables with liver detoxification properties, like bladderwrack, sea moss, kelp, dulse, and chlorella.

These things help provide all of the magnesium, potassium, and many other minerals that the body needs. As a matter of fact, Magic Moss has ninety-eight minerals that the body is made up of. Your body requires 102 minerals.

Just to give you a little reference on how great that is, the average vegan only get seventy to seventy-five minerals in their day-to-day diet. The average meat-eater only gets about fifty to sixty-five minerals in their diet. So, with us taking Magic Moss, we are getting more minerals than any other diet, structure, or plan on the planet. That is why we take it: to avoid the keto flu, keto rash, breakouts, and, next, hair falling out.

I receive questions about hair loss often. In most cases, people are not supplementing their magnesium, potassium, or electrolytes, and their hair starts to fall out. If you do not want this to happen to you, please make sure you get the magnesium potassium, and electrolytes you need.

Next, look for a positive: weight loss. On the keto diet, you can expect to lose anywhere from two to five pounds a week, which is a safe range. Any more than that, and you run the risk of losing muscle mass. We don't want to lose muscle mass, so, of course, we want to take it slow.

Ladies, if you want the nice butt, nice thighs, and to be toned, then you want to shoot for about one to three pounds of weight loss a week. Of course, the lighter you are or the less you weigh, the less weight you want to come off each week.

Here's an example if a woman weighs 150 pounds, then it's safe to say she needs to lose one pound a week or less. If a woman weighs between 150 and 200 pounds, it's safe to say that woman can lose about two pounds a week without losing or risking too much muscle loss. If a woman weighs over 200 pounds, she may lose up to five pounds a week without risking too much muscle loss.

The next thing you want to be sure to do is take pictures. I have my clients take front, side, and back photos, because the weight may go down on the scale, but your waist may be shrinking even more because this diet is so good at burning fat around the midsection. So, be sure to take "before" pictures.

I have my clients take weekly photos. Every week, on Saturdays, we take front, side, and back pictures, so we can look at side-by-side comparisons and know where the weight is coming off. And if you're gaining weight, we know where it's going on. If your waist is still shrinking but you're gaining weight, then that may be muscle. If the opposite is happening, then that is fat.

The next thing you can look for is positive signs in PCOS symptoms. Yes, that's right: this diet is great for PCOS. Anyone who is struggling with or suffering from PCOS, you also have insulin-resistance issues. The keto diet helps to not only improve but sometimes eliminate insulin resistance and PCOS altogether.

For more information on PCOS and insulin resistance plus diabetes, as well, go check out the book *The Diabetes Code* by Dr. Jason Fung. In this book, he talks about how diabetes is related to insulin resistance, and how insulin resistance is related to PCOS, and how all of this can also be related to hormone issues. If you want more of a scientific breakdown of all of this, please go check out that book.

Another good thing you can look for is clear skin, because hormones will be optimized through this diet. That means, if you have had some type of hormone manipulation or some type of hormone issues in the past, it may also have caused you to break out. Many of the women I work with who are coming off of birth control usually have hormone imbalances, and this causes their skin to break out. When they start to eat a proper diet, including all of the healthy fat you'll be eating in a keto diet, it helps with hormone production and regulation. You will notice that not only will your skin start to clear, but your hormones will optimize, as well.

Once your hormones optimize, you may notice that your sex drive goes up. You don't want to run from this, because healthy hormones are associated with a healthy sexual appetite and vice versa. If you don't have a healthy sex appetite, then you don't have healthy hormones and vice versa.

Next, you're going to also notice that your metabolic flexibility is going to improve. This means, over time, you're going to be able to burn fat and carbohydrates simultaneously. You're going to notice that when you do eat carbohydrates, it won't affect you as badly as it once did. You're not going to gain too much weight, like before. You won't hold onto those carbohydrates like you once did.

You can also expect your sleep to be much deeper and more effective. I've noticed, although a lot of times we only sleep for about six or seven hours, the deep sleep causes us to get so much good rest that we don't need any more than that. This is something you can look forward to, as well.

So, get your calories in order. Get your macros in order. Be sure to test and tweak based on the results you're getting in the mirror, from taking pictures, and from measuring your ketones on your ketone reader. Put all of this together and I promise, you're going to get some great results from this diet.

Next, we have cycling carbohydrates or cheat days. Is this something you should be doing?

Yes, but you should not be cycling in cheat days or high-carb days until you have gone through at least three months of the keto diet. This is going to assure that you are deep into ketosis, that you have achieved metabolic flexibility, and you have lost some of the fat and weight you wanted to lose.

Once you have been into ketosis and haven't cheated for about three months, you can start adding in one high-carb day. This high-carb day should still be considered a day of eating decently, which means you'll want to eat good fruits, good vegetables, and maybe have some potatoes or yams. Most of your carbohydrates on this day should still come from good, quality carbohydrates. This is not a day to have donuts, pizza, veggie burgers, etcetera. You may have beans. You may have good fruits and vegetables, potatoes, maybe some grains, and keep it there.

I'm not going to cut you off from burgers and French fries forever. Once you achieve your goal and you're down to the weight loss goal you have set for yourself, feel free to have the cheat days. Eat those burgers, fries, and, of course, the pizza. But as long as you're still attempting to lose fat or get to a certain goal, make sure you keep your cheat days or your high-carb days at a minimum and keep them clean.

If you are absolutely going to have these cheat days, I like to throw in a fasting day right after. This means, if you cheat on Saturday and you finish eating around 7:00 PM, I would have you go a full twenty-four hours before eating your keto diet again. This means you're going to go from 7:00 PM Saturday to 7:00 PM Sunday without food, only water. Then, on Sunday at 7:00 PM, you can break your fast with the high-fat fruit, like an olive or avocado or fermented vegetables. This will be sure to wipe out the excess calories you've eaten the day before and will keep you on track to losing the fat you are aiming to lose, so you get that body goal you are aiming for.

Chapter Four
Frequent Question and Answers

THIS CHAPTER IS WHERE I will break down questions and provide answers on the most popular topics I get asked.

Question #1: How do I get my protein?

My simple answer to this is, basically, how much protein do you think you need? I say this because many people, before they come over to the keto diet, have been following a traditional high-protein, high-carb, low-fat diet. Of course, once you come over to a keto state or become keto adapted, you begin to make what are called muscle-sparing ketones. Now, because you are making muscle-sparing ketones, you are also increasing human growth hormone. With these two very important things being produced in your body, protein numbers don't need to be as high. The only exception to this rule is if:

A. You are looking to body build and gain a lot of muscle.

B. If you are looking to hit a specific number based on a health issue. Maybe your doctor has told you that you needed a certain amount of protein, so they're recommending you to stick to that.

These two things are the only reasons why you should be worried about your protein intake being high. Otherwise, you should be able to get your protein numbers from your nuts, your seeds, your vegetables, and the fruits you're eating.

If you still feel the need to get more protein in, it's totally up to you to grab some hempeh, which is a meat replacement or mock meat made from hemp seeds. You may get hemp tofu or a vegan protein powder of choice. And if your body's okay with it, maybe a soy tofu or soy tempeh.

Side note: I'm not a big fan of soy, so be careful with over-consumption.

Question #2: How do I transition into a plant-based lifestyle?

This is something I'm hearing often because a lot of people are looking to go from a keto meat-based style of eating over to a vegan-keto style of eating. And, of course, the one thing I usually recommend is to keep everything plant-based. Don't come over and get caught up with the processed foods, including all the processed keto junk foods people are making now—it's still processed.

Stick to your vegetables, stick your fruits. Stick to your nuts and your seeds. As long as you're doing this, you should be just fine. Of course, coming from a meat-based diet, your protein is going to go down a little. And, of course, your carbs may come up just a little, as long as they're plant-based carbs. Keep them plant based and everything will be all right. Also, be sure to track and tweak. You should be good from there.

You can start off with your first meal of the day being plant-based, and then eat what you normally would eat for the rest of the day. Each week, eliminate one meat meal or transition one meal over to a vegan meal, if you're eating three times a day.

Week one would include one meal per day that's plant-based, and then your last two meals will be whatever you're normally eating.

Week two, your first two meals will be plant-based and your last meal of the day is still whatever you normally eat.

And then in week three, you are fully transition to all three meals each day being plant-based.

Now, if this is too short for you to adapt or too fast of a transition, of course you can slow it down. Maybe for the first month, you can eat one plant-based meal a day and two meals that are not plant-based.

Month 2: you could do two meals plant-based, and one meal not plant-based.

Month 3. Try to transition to all plant-based.

The schedule, of course, is totally up to you, however. You have to make this fit your lifestyle.

Question #3: Is the keto diet the superior diet to lose fat?

This is a great question. I get this one probably every day. I, for one, believe that yes, the keto diet is the one superior to pretty much all other diets, simply because it kills the cravings.

If you are doing a high-carbohydrate diet, a lot of times your insulin is going to be high. Which means your cravings are still going to be there for other carbohydrates. So, even if you are eating a raw, plant-based diet or if you're doing mostly fruits on your plant-based diet, you are still going to crave other carbohydrates like grains, beans, and other things that could possibly slow down weight loss, such as pizzas, veggie burgers, French fries, and other sweets.

So, what we want to do is be focused on trying to kill these cravings. This is why I say the keto diet is the better or superior diet to lose fat. Because not only are you turning from muscle glycogen (i.e., carbohydrate burning or sugar burning), you're actually going to fat burning with this diet, so you're burning more fat automatically.

Secondly, because your cravings are low and you're burning more fat, you are not limited to how you are going to eat throughout the day. This means you can go without food for sixteen hours, twenty hours, twenty-two hours, twenty-four hours, forty-eight hours—however long. And because you're burning fat, you're still losing weight, which is your goal. You are still losing the weight you want to lose, which is fat, and you're not going to be as hungry.

The reason why you won't be as hungry, is because you don't need to put in any nutrition or any carbohydrates when you're fat-adapted. Simply because you have fat on your body and because the fat is on your body, you just continue to burn that, when you're not eating.

This is why I say it's very much superior to any other diet. So, take that into consideration. And, of course, remember this is for each individual based on their goals and their needs and their wants.

Question #4: How many carbs should I eat?

It's totally up to you based on, of course, your genetics, your current state, plus whether or not you're able to digest and utilize carbohydrates efficiently or not. For a lot of people, I usually have them start around forty to fifty grams total of carbohydrates, and then we tweak from there.

If we get you into ketosis with forty or fifty grams and you feel like you want a little bit more, we slowly add ten to twenty grams of carbs per week and see if we remain in ketosis. If you add ten or twenty grams of carbs on week two and you stay in ketosis, great.

If you need a little bit more carbs or you feel like you want more, try adding a few more of plant-based carbs, say ten to twenty grams more. If you're still in ketosis, once again add ten to twenty more. Basically, you're going to stop either when you're satisfied with the amount of carbs you're eating or when you begin to drop your ketone levels or you get kicked out of ketosis overall.

This is how we do it. This is why we test and tweak, test and tweak. Every time we meet a certain number, we tweak it. If it's not something that won't work, it's not ideal. Once it's ideal, we stop there and continue on with those amounts.

Question #5: Will I gain the weight back when I go back to carbs?

People fall prey to this with all diets. People start to do a diet, they go for two, three, four months, and then they go right back to eating the way they once ate. And guess what? You start to gain your weight back.

Why is this? Well, simply, because you can't go too fast on any diet. If I'm coming from a 2000-calorie diet and I start back eating 3000 calories all of a sudden, eventually I'm going to gain all of my weight back plus some, in most cases.

How do we avoid gaining weight back? Whether or not you're keto, whether or not you are high carb, when you lose your weight, you want to do what's called reverse dieting, which means, once you hit your goal weight or once you get to a point where you're absolutely happy with the result. Maybe, if it's not your goal weight, you're just happy where you are.

You can't just jump back into eating how you want. You have to slowly introduce things back in, just like we introduce the diet slowly into our lifestyle. You want to take it slow. As a matter of fact, when you're trying to reverse that, you want to go even slower.

So, for instance, some of the things I do for my clients is add 100 calories back to her diet once a week. Okay. If you're eating 1500 calories right now, this week you're going to do 1600; next week, you're going to do 1700; and the following week, you're going to do 1800.

This is something that not many trainers and not many nutritionists are doing. As a matter of fact, the average person doesn't even know to do this. It is very important that you reverse diet, if you want to keep your results.

That means carbohydrates, as well. If you're eating 100 grams of carbohydrates on your keto diet and you want to slowly transition back to higher carbs, then what you want to do is maybe add twenty grams of carbs each week to your diet.

Yes, it is mundane. Yes, it sucks for most people, because they don't want to keep track of this, which of course is why most people just hire a coach to do it. But if you don't have the money for a coach or you don't want to pay the money for your coach, then you have to take the time out and do it, if you want to keep your results.

Slowly add back in the carbs, twenty grams at a time. Yes, this should get you roughly under 100 calories a week. Twenty grams of carbs is right about 80 calories a week. What that means basically you're going to be adding 80 calories a week until you get to the ideal number of carbs you want. I have to warn you that as you go back to a higher-carb diet, you must also drop the fats. If you're adding twenty grams of carbs per week, you must be dropping the fat by ten to twenty grams of fat a week, as well.

> Week one would look like this: 150 grams of fat, 100 grams of carbs.

> Week two would look like this: 130 grams of fat and 120 grams of carbs.

> Week three would look like this: 110 grams of fat and 160 grams of carbs.

And you just continue to move these numbers slowly over time, until you at least get where you want or where you feel comfortable. Then you can stop there and get back to your normal diet.

Question #6: Can I eat beans on this diet?

Well, most beans of course are not going to be very compatible with this diet. But, like I tell all of my clients, as long as it fits your macros, I'm totally okay with you doing that. The reason why I say that is because, I have clients right now who are eating lentils and adding chickpeas to their keto diets, and they are still in ketosis. If this is something you want to get into, just make sure you track your calories. Because beans do have good fiber in them, so you should be fine. It should buffer out the carbs you are eating.

You just can't have an overabundance of beans. Personally, I'm going to suggest that you stick to chickpeas, black beans, lentils, and peas. Everything else, I would be wary or cautious about adding to the diet.

Question #7: Is keto safe for diabetics?

I'm pretty sure I get this question two to three times a day, just because diabetes is very prevalent in this country. Keto is definitely safe for diabetics, especially if you have diabetes 2.

I have noticed that this diet dramatically helps with Type 2 diabetes. Even for Type 1 diabetes, it works just fine, because you limit the amount of insulin you need to produce since you aren't eating many foods that have a lot of sugar. This diet has been helpful for my clients with both types of diabetes, and me as well, because I once had diabetes, too.

For more information on diabetes and a deeper dive into keto diet and fasting, please go check out the book, **The Diabetes Code** by Dr. Jason Fung.

Question #8: Where do you get your omega-3s?

Omega-3s are all in the high-fat diet. You can get these omega-3s from your seeds, like hemp seeds, chia seeds, flax seeds. You can also get omega-3s from some of your sea vegetables. Some seaweeds, sea moss, and bladderwrack have omega-3s, as well. And overall, if you want more omega-3s, you can also dive into avocados.

Question #9: Can I gain weight on a vegan keto diet?

Absolutely, you can gain weight. The simple equation for that is to eat more in a caloric surplus. Then you will definitely gain muscle. I must be honest here, though, this is not the easiest way to gain muscle, because when it comes to gaining muscle or gaining more weight, you do want an insulin response. An insulin response comes from more carbohydrates.

You can slowly come out of the keto diet and go more into a cyclical keto diet. Basically, what this would mean is you do three or four days in keto to stay pretty lean, and then the other two to three days you would actually go in and have high carbs on those days. This could help you bulk up to get that insulin response while simultaneously keeping you fairly lean by doing the keto diet and staying metabolically flexible from burning both carbs and fats.

Question #9: Does a vegan diet consist of mostly carbs?

The traditional vegan diet that we know does, yes. It consists of many, many carbs, and, as a matter of fact, when people go vegan, they already don't understand or know how to go vegan. They just eat what they think they have access to, and this tends to be heavy carbs.

The reason for this is because they are convenient—everything is carbs. You have beans, you have rice, you have other legumes, and, of course, grains. All of your fruits and vegetables are mostly carbs. And then you also have lots of not-so-good vegan foods like veggie burgers and pizza. These are all carbohydrates.

Many vegans don't necessarily focus on their health. They're just attempting to stay away from animal products. So, in a lot of cases, what I do to get my point across is I make a joke and say, "Hey, if you're sitting at a table and you're vegan and the table doesn't have any animal products, that table is good to eat!"

However, most of you are here to lose weight, to protect your health, or to fix or improve some type of health issue you may have. We cannot eat all of those processed foods, all the junk foods, all of the so-called "vegan foods." We have to focus on plant-based sources.

We have many ways of approaching this. When people do a raw, fruitarian diet, some people do mostly raw diet with just raw fruits and vegetables. Some people do an overall plant-based diet, where they allow some cook foods. And now that you've read this book, of course, you also have another option.

For my people who don't do well digesting carbohydrates, you have a keto route as well.

Question #10: Can I have soy or mock meats?

When I create a lot of nutrition plans for my clients, I may add in one or two meat replacements just because it's a little more convenient. These meat replacements, are hempeh, which is a hemp-seed meat replacement made with hemp seeds and peanuts. This is a replacement also for tempeh, which is made from soy. My clients love it. They do well with it. They add a little sauce to it, cut it up, cook it, and it's amazing.

Also, I suggest hemp tofu. This is tofu made from hemp seeds. If you look up the history of tofu, it actually originated as hemp tofu before it became soy tofu. This is a very long history and you will have to do some digging for it, but it is there.

This is what I suggest. Of course, if you are someone who does well with soy, you may have tofu or tempeh from soy, too.

I personally don't recommend it for myself or my clients, because we want to stay away from soy, just in case it does cause any hormone-imbalance issues. I have noticed that soy does to me and many of my clients. Although I won't recommend it, I will not tell you not to eat soy. You must make this choice on your own.

Question #11: Is vegan keto sustainable long-term?

Of course, I am going to say yes, it's sustainable long-term! However, I don't think it's something everyone should do long-term.

I look at a vegan keto diet as a fix-the-issue type of diet before slowly transitioning back into eating more fruits and vegetables that are a little bit higher in carbs. What do I mean by this? Most people eat themselves into a certain place, like insulin resistance, PCOS diabetes and other things, like hormone imbalances.

Because we have eaten our way into these diets, this lets me know we have been eating improperly for an extended period of time, which means it's going to take something just as extreme on the other side to get us out of it. This is where we start to feed the body the keto diet, to fix some of these issues.

Once we get the weight off and once we get the insulin resistance taken care of, we slowly reverse diet our way back to eating more fruits and vegetables, and upping those cards. Now, I don't suggest just dropping keto all at once. Once again, I suggest you reverse diet out of it. Some people do keto for about three months; some people do six months. The longest I've seen my clients do is nine months.

Once we reach our goals and we feel that we're okay, I slowly start to bump up their carbs and their calories, so they can get more into a healthier, sustainable route. And when I say healthier, I mean mentally healthier, because many people, after three, six, or nine months, they mentally start to feel like they want more options, even if they have so many options inside keto.

To return you to mental health or ease after six or nine months, if that's all you need, then yes, we slowly start to implement more fruits into your diet. And we raise the carbs, just like I talked about above. As we raise the carbs, we want to lower the fat. This is how we transition out of the vegan keto diet.

Question #13: Do you get bored with food choices?

Of course. This is what I was talking about in the last question. Yes, you're going to get bored with your food choices, especially if you're someone like me who eats the same things every day. I personally don't like to do a lot of work or put a lot of thought process into what I'm eating. I eat the same things every day.

However, even though there are so many choices of foods you can eat, but you still are going to get bored, but not because there are not a lot of food choices. You're going to get bored because there are a lot more food choices *outside* of the diet. You're going to get bored of not being able to eat more fruit. You're going to get bored of not being able to eat a lot of your sweet potatoes, potatoes, things like that. You're going to get bored of not having those nice cheat meals like the veggie burgers, French fries, pizza, and vegan donuts.

This is what's going to make it boring, because many of you are currently eating like that now. Getting rid of the donuts and the pizza and the veggie burgers is going to be hard for you. And, of course, it's going to be boring.

But this is not a keto thing. This is a diet thing, period. If you were to do a high-carb diet, you're still going to have to get rid of the veggie burgers, pizza, and French fries, if you want to lose weight. On a high-carb diet, you have to follow more fruits and vegetables still. Either way it goes, yes, it's going to be a little more boring than what I call your "freedom diet."

A Freedom Diet basically means you're free to eat whatever you want. If that's the type of diet you're on now, I don't care what kind of lifestyle you choose to follow to lose weight, you are going to have to cut things out of your freedom diet. Even if you eat meat, you're still going to have to stick to regular meats like chicken breasts, plus fish and vegetables. This is usually how it works on the eating side.

If you go over to the high-carb vegan side, you're going to have to do fruits, vegetables, and maybe some legumes. Everything else, you're going to have to stay away from, like the veggie burgers and the comfort foods, just like you are going to have to when it comes to keto.

So, all of these diets are "boring," because you can't have those freedom foods you often have. But we're just trying to get to a goal. You want to hurry up and get there, because the quicker you get there, the quicker you can get back to your freedom foods.

Question #14: Can I eat fruit on this diet?

Yes, you can. You likely know this answer: I don't care what you eat, as long as you follow your macros and your calories. Something I tell a lot of my clients, though, is if you're going to mess around with some other things, stay at or under the calories you've set for yourself. Stay at or under the carbs limit you are set to eat.

As long as you do that, you can slowly add in certain fruits, like berries—raspberries, blueberries, blackberries. These do not kick you out of ketosis as long as you eat them in moderation. But you don't want to eat too many of them.

Things like cantaloupe, honeydew, and even seeded watermelon also will not kick you out of ketosis, so you may have some of these melons. Again, in moderation: you can't eat too many of them.

You can also eat other things such as olives and avocados, which are fruits. You can also eat jackfruit. These are not super-sweet, so you can get away with eating them within your macros. Just generally be careful with how many fruits you eat. I recommend you enjoy them and then get back to your diet.

Question #15: Why should I soak my nuts and seeds?

A lot of you hear me talk about soaking your nuts and seeds. It's very important to soak your nuts and your seeds because we need to activate them.

What does that mean to activate them? If you leave nuts or seeds sitting on the shelf for years, a lot of times they will not spoil or rot. They will look the same for the most part. Activating your nuts and seeds activates the enzymes. What am I talking about here? With activated nuts and seeds, if you leave these sitting out for a week, they will go bad. The reason behind this is because you have activated the enzymes.

You want to activate enzymes simply because we should be eating foods with enzymes in them, so we get proper digestion. Not only that, if you don't soak your nuts or your seeds, you'll eat what we call enzyme inhibitors that are found in nuts and seeds. Some people may also point out phytates, which are also in the nuts and seeds. These enzyme inhibitors slow down digestion. So, if you haven't been eating a lot of nuts and seeds and you're constipated, this is where you want to look, too. These un-activated nuts and seeds are usually a big piece behind constipation, especially for people who eat a lot of them.

So, soak your nuts and seeds, anywhere from four hours to eight hours. Some people can even let them go a little bit longer. I've seen people soak their nuts and seeds for twenty-four hours. I usually recommend you put them in to soak before bed and by the time you wake up, your nuts and seeds will be ready for you to eat.

Question #16: Why do I get constipated on keto diet?

Once again, this goes right back to soaking those nuts and seeds. Many people who become constipated on a keto diet are also eating a lot of nuts and seeds and/or nut butter. Many of the nut butters you come by will not be made from sprouted or soaked nuts. They are made from just plain old dry almonds or peanuts or whatever, so it's just dry nuts being made into butter. What this means is it still has the enzyme inhibitors. It still has everything we talked about that is going to cause some of those digestive issues for you.

Make sure you are soaking your nuts and seeds. Now, people are getting hip to sprouting their nuts and seeds before making it into a butter. You can definitely can find pre-made almond butter that has been sprouted. You can also find pumpkin seed butter that has been sprouted and many other sprouted nuts and seed butters.

Not only that, many people go over to the keto diet extremely too fast. What happens is your body has not built the enzymes to break down all of the fats you begin putting into your body. So, to counteract that, look into getting a great enzyme supplement to help you to break down these new fats.

Remember: you have been breaking down carbohydrates at a high rate for ten, twenty, thirty, forty, even fifty years. This sudden shift to higher fats is going to be pretty rough on your body. Your body is not used to it. Your body doesn't know what it's doing, and it's asking you, "Why are you giving me this? I don't know what it is."

In that case, for the first few weeks and months, maybe even the first three months, you want to make sure you're getting in some enzymes before you eat anything. Thirty minutes before you have your meal, take an enzyme or two. That will help to break down the fats. As long as you're doing this plus soaking your nuts and seeds, you should be good to go.

Question #17: Is it healthy for ketones to be in your blood?

Yes. And as a matter of fact, it's beneficial and it should be for everybody. The reason why I say that is, even if you do not go all the way over to a keto diet, you should at least be practicing some form of fasting. The body was made to fast. Ketones are great for the brain. Ketones are great for the body, and, actually, it is great to be metabolically flexible. This means the body burns carbs *and* fats for energy.

Once upon a time, back when you were a child and felt your greatest, you had all that child energy. You were metabolically flexible, because you were eating the fat, especially if you were breastfed. You were getting breast milk from your mother, which is a very high-fat type formula, and also you were getting carbohydrates as you were raised. You were metabolically flexible, because you were getting both and able to burn both.

Bottom line: even if you do not do the keto diet, you should at least be fasting. These are both great and therapeutic for the body. Definitely try that out and get you some ketones in your blood.

Question #18: Can I transition to keto while breastfeeding?

I've worked with many, many, many mothers—expectant mothers, mothers who are breastfeeding—and each and every time, I let them know my opinion: No, I do not suggest you transition or change your diet in the middle of a pregnancy or while you are still breastfeeding. The reason why I say this is because the body is very resilient, but it's set in its ways.

It's used to eating a certain type of way and used to building and utilizing the nutrients you have been given, so trying to make an extreme switch in the middle of breastfeeding or in the middle of pregnancy can be very harmful to the body. I definitely *do not suggest* you do that, not until you're done breastfeeding.

Also, the reason why I do not suggest making any dramatic switches or changes in the body while you're doing your breastfeeding is because the female body wants all of the nutrients. It doesn't want to give up any nutrients while it's pregnant or breastfeeding a child. When you're breastfeeding and/or trying to grow another human, you want to give it proper, equal amounts of protein, carbs, and fats. You don't want to cut down on any of them because a mother needs to be giving her child an equal, balanced amount of nutrients.

Question #19: What are nightshades and should I be staying away from them?

A nightshade is a type of plant that can give some people negative side effects. Nightshades have been a pretty big topic during the few last few years. I actually agree with some of these points raised.

Do you stay away from them? Maybe not. Maybe you just cut down on them, even though some of these nightshades are very hard to stay away from. If you feel like you can stay totally away from these nightshades, fine. Please do that. But I do suggest at least cutting down on the nightshades.

That includes the following list:

- ✓ Goji berries
- ✓ Eggplant
- ✓ Bell peppers
- ✓ Chili peppers
- ✓ Paprika
- ✓ Potatoes, not including the sweet potato
- ✓ Tomatoes
- ✓ Tomatillos

These are nightshades. Once again, if you cannot totally stay away from them, at least cut down on how many you include in your diet.

Question #20: What are good keto snacks?

These are a few snacks you can get away with on the vegan keto diet:

❖ Almond or nut crackers: there are plenty of nut crackers out there. Just find the best one and have those on hand for snacks.

❖ Add MCT oil to your coffee.

❖ Coconut cream or coconut milk with berries. This is something me and my clients have been using for years. We call them coconut berries, and they're an amazing, satisfying quick snack.

❖ Avocado with salt and pepper

❖ Pickles

❖ Kale chips

❖ Chia-seed pudding

❖ Flax crackers

❖ Pumpkin seeds

- ❖ Sunflower seeds
- ❖ Olives
- ❖ Seaweed snacks
- ❖ Any nut butter of choice

Once again, for all of the above, if the snack involves nuts and seeds, please do your best to soak or sprout them. If you're going to buy them from someone who is providing them, try to find sources that include pre-soaked nut butter or soaked nuts and seeds, also known as sprouted.

Question #21: How should I work out to maximize fat loss?

The way the human body is made, and the way many of us should be operating, is to be moving every day. In that case, I usually suggest you get up and move every day. Thirty minutes minimum. This can be walking, this can be strength training. Of course, if you want to get really extreme with it, I do have a small section with a chart that talks about how much you should be doing with strength training, how much you should be doing with cardio, etc., etc.

But if you want faster results with your weight loss, you definitely should be doing some form of cardio or weight training for thirty minutes a day at least five times a week. Personally, I think you should work out every day, but some people don't have that luxury. So, I say be sure to work out at least five times a week for thirty minutes a day.

And like I said, working out can be just a walk. I usually recommend a minimum of two miles a day for a lot of my clients, because the body was meant to walk for extended periods or extended distances. We may not be able or have the time to do ten or twenty miles, like our ancestors once walked, but do at least two miles a day. If you're moving at a decent pace, you can get two miles done in thirty minutes.

Definitely get walking. This is going to be something huge if you're looking to lose the weight fast. If you need to take more time to walk your two miles, that's totally fine. Just get it in. This is going to be very helpful.

Conclusion & Warning

I WANT YOU TO KNOW this: no one should diet or remain in the caloric deficit inside of ketosis or even calorie counting for an extended period of time. My suggestion to many of my clients is to diet for about eight to twelve weeks and then have a diet break for four to six weeks. Then, you may go right back into your diet.

One big reason why I warn you against dieting too long or staying in ketosis too long or even calorie counting too long is simply because I've seen many people, including very famous body builders, physique competitors, and others who are doing an extended period of caloric restriction, ketosis, or even calorie counting, who often have health issues, such as hormonal issues, which of course leads to a lack of sexual stamina and potential erectile dysfunction.

Women can develop issues such as a menstrual cycle that is painful or lasts longer. Some women, once they get too lean or after they have been dieting too long, even have periods that go away. This usually causes women to get in the cycle of only having a menstrual cycle once or twice a year. Some women skip an entire year.

This often happens, once again, with people who diet too long, who don't cycle their dieting correctly, and who are in a caloric deficit or who restrict carbohydrates for too long. I personally think that everyone should hire a professional or a coach to help them with this. Someone who knows about regulating hormones through manipulating calories, as I am describing to you now.

If you are not familiar with this, I definitely advise you hire a coach. Of course, if you'd like me to be your coach, I would love to work with you.

You can email me at info@iamthevegantrainer.com or you can simply DM (direct message) me on Instagram.

You can find me on Instagram here:

@IamTheVeganTrainer

Once again, I would love to work with you and love to give you the guidance and coaching you need so you maintain a healthy hormonal system or healthy menstrual cycle. If you're going through menopause, I can help you to have a healthy menopause, as well.

I hope you've enjoyed this book. I thank you for reading. I thank you for supporting and showing the love you have shown thus far. And I can't wait to bring you the next book.

Vegan keto has taken me far, putting me in sight of my goals and my clients in sight of their goals. When done correctly, we get to reach our goals and then slowly start to implement fruits and other carbs, healthy carbs, back into our diets. This keeps the natural flow of the body going, and, of course, this is how men and women should be eating.

Once again, to wrap this up, I want you to know that the neither the Vegan Keto Diet or the regular Keto Diet, for meat-eaters, are not something you should live on for the rest of your life. This is simply a means to an end. You want to fix some of the issues we have, such as insulin resistance, diabetes, PCOS, etc. Once these things are fixed and/or starting to improve, then we want to slowly start to add healthy carbohydrates back in to our diets, such as fruits, more vegetables, and of course beans and healthy grains.

I may talk more about this in my next book, so definitely stay tuned. Until then, continue to be healthy and remember, I love you.

TAY SWEAT

A Complete Keto Guide

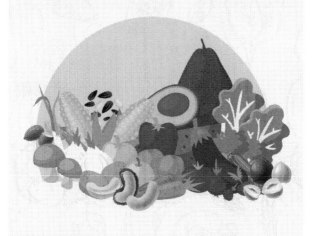

A Complete Keto Guide

How to Eat Keto – Your Keto Kitchen

Vegetables

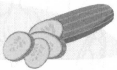

Alfalfa sprouts
Artichokes
Arugula
Asparagus
Bean sprouts
Beets
Bok choy
Broccoli
Broccoli sprouts
Broccolini

Brussel sprouts
Cabbage, red
or green
Cauliflower
Celery
Chard
Chives
Collard greens
Cucumber

Endive
Ginger
Kale
Kelp
Leeks
Lettuce
Mushrooms
Nori
Okra

Olives
Radishes
Rhubarb
Rutabaga
Scallions
Seaweed or
sea moss

Herbs & Spices

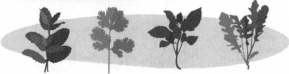

Allspice
Anise
Basil
Bay leaf
Bladder wrack
Burdock root
Cardamom
Celery seed
Chlorella
Cilantro
Cinnamon
Clove

Coriander
Cumin
Dandelion root
Dill
Dulse
Fennel
Garlic
Ginger
Horseradish
Juniper
Juniper berry
Lavender

Lemon balm
Maca
Mace
Milk thistle
Mint
Mustard
Nutmeg
Oregano
Parsley
Peppercorn
Pine Pollen

Poppy seed
Rosemary
Sage
Sea salt
Sesame seed
Tongkat ali
Turmeric
Vanilla bean

HOW TO VEGAN KETO

Fats

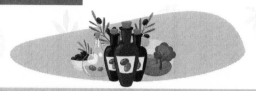

Almond milk
Almond oil
Almond yogurt
Avocado oil
Coconut cream
Coconut meat
Coconut milk

Coconut oil
Coconut yogurt
Flax seed oil
Hazelnut oil
Hemp seed oil

Macadamia nut oil
MCT oil
Olive oil
Palm kernel oil
Walnut oil

Liquids

Almond milk
Coconut milk
Coconut water
Coffee - no added sugar

Green juice – with no fruit or added sugar

Kombucha - no added sugar

Sweeteners

Monk Fruit
Stevia
Xylitol

Seeds

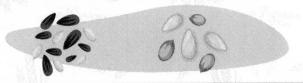

Chia
Flax
Hemp
Poppy
Pumpkin

Sesame
Sunflower
Watermelon

Nuts

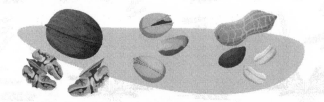

Almond
Brazil
Cashews - eat sparingly
Hazelnut
Macadamia

Peanut - eat sparingly
Pecan
Pistachio
Tiger
Walnut

Fruits

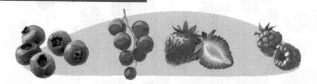

Ackee - can be
found in the
Caribbean
Avocado
Blackberry
Blueberry
Cantaloupe
Clementine
Grapefruit
Honeydew

Melon
Jackfruit
Kiwi
Orange
Olive
Papaya
Passion fruit
Pineapple

Raspberry
Strawberry
Watermelon

*All fruits and melons
must have seeds

Base rules to follow

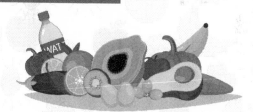

1. Eat plant-based foods only.
2. Keep carbs between 40-200 grams. Determine your optimal amount by starting with 40 grams of carbs, then slowly working your way up until you are kicked out of ketosis. Check your ketones to make sure you are on the right path. Once you are out of ketosis, you know that you've eaten too many carbs.
3. Eat more healthy fats than carbs and protein.
4. Eat when you are hungry or outside of your fasting window.
5. Do not starve yourself.
6. Work out at least three to four times a week.

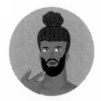

Weight Training

Weight training is something that most people should be doing, but are not.

Weight Training Tips

Of the people who are doing it, about 70% of them are doing it incorrectly. If you need coaching on how to do this the correct way, visit my webpage at **iamthevegantrainer.com**

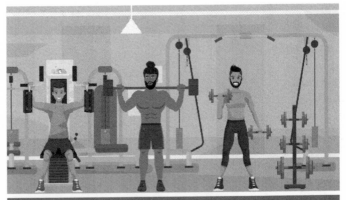

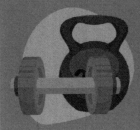

Weight training should be done three to five times a week, depending on your goals. If your goal is to lose fat while also building or toning your muscle, you should be doing cardio and weight training on the same day.

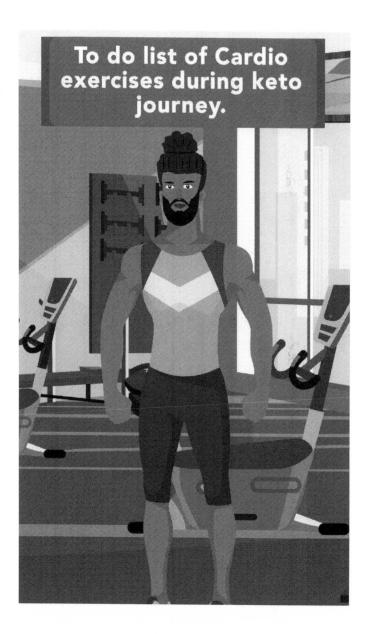

To do list of Cardio exercises during keto journey.

Cardio

You should be doing at least 30 minutes of cardio, four to six times a week (depending on your goals).

Cardio Exercises & Machines

Jump rope, treadmill, walk or run, swimming, dancing, elliptical, boxing or kickboxing, skating, rowing machine, cycling.

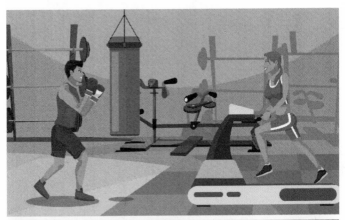

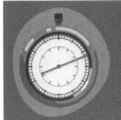

Cardio = Anything that can get your heart rate to 130 beats per minute. You should aim for this heart rate for 20-30 minutes.

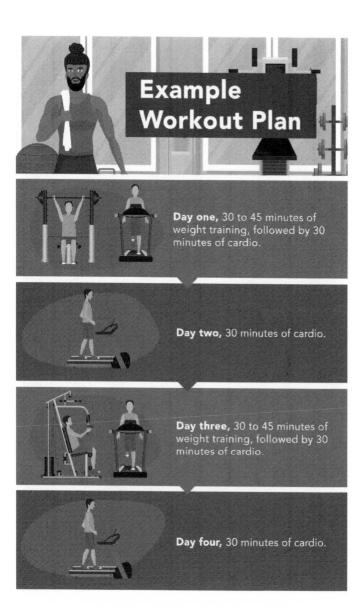

Example Workout Plan

Day one, 30 to 45 minutes of weight training, followed by 30 minutes of cardio.

Day two, 30 minutes of cardio.

Day three, 30 to 45 minutes of weight training, followed by 30 minutes of cardio.

Day four, 30 minutes of cardio.

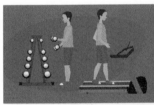

Day five, 30 to 45 minutes of weight training, followed by 30 minutes of cardio.

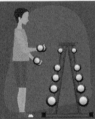

Day six, which is Saturday 30 which is usually a day you're going to be eating a little bit more because this is your day of social activity in our society. This day should look like 30 to 45 minutes of weight training, followed by 30 minutes of cardio.

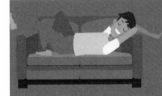

Day seven, rest.

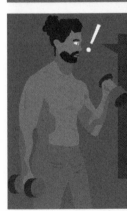

This workout plan is aggressive and is designed for someone who wants to achieve his or her goals at a fast pace. Feel free to adjust the intensity of this plan to your specific goals. The exercises you should be doing will vary. I did not include specific exercises in this plan, because I want everyone to be safe. Please hire a coach or trainer to help with this part of your journey.

Acknowledgments

I FIRST WOULD LIKE to start off by thanking my wife, Whitney Lee Sweat, for all of the love, the sacrificing, and the support she's done and given for us. This book is not only mine. This is book is just as much hers, based on all the love and hard work she's put into me, the book, and everything in between.

I would also like to thank my best friend, Edward Henley, for all of the great conversations we've had about writing books, becoming better men, and being pillars for our community, for our culture, for our race, for our country, and for those who come from areas like we once came from.

I'd also like to acknowledge all of my supporters, whether it's from Instagram, YouTube, Facebook, a VegFest. I love you all, and I will continue to pour everything I have, all of my energy, into you all, because you are the ones who keep me going. You are the ones who make me get up out of bed every morning to make the videos, continue to study, read, further my education, and get credentialed. It's you who pushed me to be who I am today. So, I'd like to thank you and let you know this book would not be possible without you, as well.

About Tay

TAY SWEAT is a plant-based nutritionist and lecturer who goes by the name the Vegan Trainer. He is currently helping thousands of people lose fat, gain lean muscle, and reclaim their health with his online programs and community. He is the author of *The Wild Rabbit* and is working on another book for plant-based athletes. *STAY TUNED!*

Visit www.IAmtheVeganTrainer.com

Follow me on my Instagram: @iamthevegantrainer

On Facebook, check me out at:

facebook.com/taysweatvegantrainer

Made in the USA
Middletown, DE
14 February 2019